TYPE 2 DIABETES?

Break Free Naturally, with Hintonia

Terry Lemerond
and
Jacob Teitelbaum, M.D.

The purpose of this book is to educate. It is not intended to serve as a replacement for professional medical advice. Any use of the information in this book is at the reader's discretion. This book is sold with the understanding that neither the publisher nor the author has any liability or responsibility for any injury caused or alleged to be caused directly or indirectly by the information contained in this book. While every effort has been made to ensure its accuracy, the book's contents should not be construed as medical advice. To obtain medical advice on your individual health needs, please consult a qualified healthcare practitioner.

TYPE 2 DIABETES?
Break Free Naturally, with Hintonia

www.TTNPublishing.com

Library of Congress Control Number: 2020922200
Print ISBN: 978-1-952507-10-6
eBook ISBN: 978-1-952507-09-0

Editor: Michele Olson
Design: Larry Bower
Formatting: Alt 19 Creative

Printed in the United States of America

This book is dedicated to all the true health seekers in the world.

Contents

CHAPTER 1
You Are In Charge—And Here Is Why You Need to Be!

Yes, you *are* in charge. You're always in charge of your health, despite the healthcare system trying to convince you that your health is dependent on your doctor.

Here's the simple truth: Your doctor is simply one health consultant available to you, offering minimal tools relative to the whole healthcare toolkit. For diabetes, except for insulin for childhood diabetes (Type 1—more on diabetes types later) and metformin, most of the medications offered to lower blood sugar have historically caused more harm than good.

But most physicians, well-meaning as they are, don't take the time to look into the research showing the toxicity of these medications. They only see what is spoon-fed to them by the drug companies.

Physicians' education after medical school is almost entirely paid for by drug companies. Sadly, despite being good, well-meaning institutions and people, even the med schools and professors are now hooked on drug money. What we are told is "Evidence-Based Medicine

(EBM)" often turns out to be rubbish, after an objective analysis of the data. This is why Dr. Marcia Angell, M.D., a past editor of the *New England Journal of Medicine* (*NEJM*) has said that she doesn't believe much of what she reads in journals anymore.

For example, standard medical training excludes virtually all-natural options! Physicians are taught that almost all of these are quackery. Doctors feel they don't even have to look at the research, because conventional wisdom says it is all "pseudoscience."

So when it comes to natural options, most physicians sadly are like members of the worst kinds of religious cults. They suffer from what essentially is a toxic and blinding form of mind control expertly woven by a financially, heavily entrenched "healthcare" system.

Doctors will doubt this, but ask your doctor one simple question, "Who pays for the journals you read and the conferences you attend?" (Hint: Drug and medical product companies.) Ask your healthcare professionals if they have seen the research showing that studies paid for by drug companies are likely to be simply unbelievable.

Translation: Almost all the "research" doctors read, which guides their prescribing, is slick advertising masquerading as science.

We want to stress this: Your doctors, people in the pharmaceutical industry and FDA, and pretty much everyone else we've met in the healthcare system, are well-meaning folks who think they are doing the right thing. But they are hardly the people we would approach for accurate information.

Abdicating the power to make your healthcare choices to your doctor can be a really bad idea. Instead, use your doctor as a consultant. But at the end of the day, *you* are the boss of your life and health.

The good news? There are strong movements afoot in the healthcare industry to decrease some of the influence of drug money. But this is going to require time to take hold. Meanwhile, education is power. Using the best of natural and standard treatments, diabetes can be safely and effectively treated. And in fact, diabetes becomes optional.

Our goals in this book:

1. To give you the background to better understand diabetes so you can make effective choices.
2. To teach you the research about a remarkably helpful herbal, called *Hintonia latiflora*, which can markedly improve your diabetes, often even making it go away!

So are you ready to become the informed boss of your healthcare? Ready for diabetes to be optional? **Then let's start!**

DIABETES *IS* OPTIONAL

When it comes to diabetes, you might think it's inevitable that you'll eventually get this terrible disease. But it's not inevitable. Not at all. We're here to tell you why.

In today's world, you undoubtedly know someone with diabetes. Maybe you even know several people, perhaps family members, with diabetes. And maybe you've even been diagnosed with "prediabetes" or diabetes itself.

Diabetes was once a rare disease, but today it is disturbingly common. The Centers for Disease Control and Prevention (CDC for short) tell us that 12.2% of American adults and 192,000 children under the age of 20 have Type 2 diabetes. One in three American adults now have prediabetes (more about that later). And it's projected that one in three of us will have full-blown, Type 2 diabetes by 2050, nearly tripling the current rate.

Until just a couple of decades ago, Type 2 diabetes was called "adult-onset diabetes." The disease was virtually unheard of in people under 50. Now, no thanks to our Standard American Diet (SAD) and our general lack of enthusiasm for exercise, Type 2 diabetes is a disease of all ages and growing alarmingly common in our Big-Mac-fed couch potato children.

A PERSONAL STORY OUR FRIEND KATHLEEN SHARED WITH US

I was recently marching in a parade with a group of friends. Among us was a little girl, about 10 years old. She came up to me and announced, "I don't understand parades."

I asked, "What don't you understand about parades?"

She replied (I am not kidding you): "Why would we be out here when we could be at home on the couch watching TV?"

I pointed out that it was a perfect fall day. There were large crowds of real people, not TV people, and she could wave and say "hi" to them.

"There are real people on TV," she rebounded.

"But you can't talk to them or interact with them. These are your neighbors. Isn't that fun?" I asked.

"No," she concluded, crossing her arms defiantly in front of her slightly chubby chest.

She spent the parade (with her mom's permission) riding in a car that accompanied us carrying several people who were disabled.

I watched her with sadness, knowing that in a few years, she will probably be one of thousands of teenagers with diabetes.

Here's a thought for those who are on the north side of 50. What if age is meaningless? It is! What if 50 is the new 30 and 70 is the new 45?

It can be!

Right now, Americans are living longer. You can live longer too, if you make the right choices. For the first time in history, the life expectancy of our children may be lower than the life expectancy of our generation. This disturbing news is a direct effect of the lifestyle choices they are being taught.

We all have a choice. You have a choice. That American myth about aging, that "aging isn't for sissies," is nonsense. Those myths are largely devised to sell stuff—OTC drugs for acid reflux, sleep aids, pain pills and a wide range of pharmaceuticals, including prescription drugs to treat depression, heart disease, cancer, erectile dysfunction, weak bladders and yes, diabetes.

We have the tools at our disposal to lead long and healthy lives if we take care of ourselves. Taking care of ourselves means enjoying fun and pleasure. For example, chocolate is a health food!

So, our simple goal is to have you live a long and healthy life and to die young at a ripe old age.

Put simply, there is no need to stop the clock. We'll all collect years and experience over time. But being *old* is optional. We firmly believe that all of us can live a healthy 120 years or more, while feeling like we are in our 30s.

TUNE-UPS

From Dr. Teitelbaum: *Do you give your car tune-ups? My car has over 100,000 miles on it, but I spend a little cash and a little time every year to give it a tune-up. Because of this, it feels and runs like a brand-new car.*

If I hadn't done the basic maintenance over the years, it would unnecessarily feel like an old car. People age in the same way.

Most people have never ever had a tune-up. Not even once! Instead, they've had "checkups", where they go in regularly to see if they have "IT" yet ("IT" being some expensive-to-treat illness). But when was the last time the doctor actually did something to optimize function and how you feel, instead of just masking symptoms or treating acute problems?

Meanwhile, research over the last two years has suggested that most cancer screening may have caused more harm than good. Although there is a place for these tests, when used to screen otherwise healthy people they become toxic. These include many prostate, breast, thyroid and other cancer screens.

So, IMHO, (In my humble opinion), the preventive screening tests that are worth doing are:

1. Checking blood pressure and blood sugar
2. Colonoscopy every 10 years beginning at age 50
3. Eye pressure screening for glaucoma every few years

There's not much left for a yearly checkup. I have come to the point that except for these screenings, I largely recommend that if people are feeling well and not having any suspicious symptoms, they should stay away from physicians.

THE NEW BREED OF PHYSICIANS

Although standard medicine is a dinosaur heading toward a cliff's edge, we don't have to go with it. Thousands of physicians are expanding their horizons, expanding their "healthcare toolkits" and immersing themselves in what scientific research and clinical experience really shows.

As they do this, they find their ability to help blossoms. They feel like they have "woken up." They fall under the names "Holistic Physicians" or "Naturopathic Doctors." They can be found at many medical society web sites including:

TuneUpDocs.com
Naturopathic.org

These doctors are learning how to not only cure illness, but also to optimize health. When we have learned to optimize health expertly, illness will become more and more irrelevant.

GETTING A TUNE-UP

Begin the process of optimizing your health by getting a tune-up. This can be done for free with a 10-minute quiz available at TuneUpDocs.com. The quiz can even evaluate key labs, if available. Basically, it will assess 12 key areas of health, including sleep, pain, hormones, immunity, nutrition, digestion, optimizing metabolism and energy, etc.

OPTIMIZING BLOOD SUGAR LEVELS

As we have mentioned, diabetes is optional. Start with a few key lifestyle tips:

1. Avoid excess sugar dumped into food.
We get 18% of our calories from the 140 pounds of sugar a year dumped into each of our diets in food processing. This doesn't mean you can't enjoy sweets. We love pampering that sweet tooth! You just need to do so healthfully. My book, *A Complete Guide to Beating Sugar Addiction,* will show you how to keep the pleasure—healthfully.

2. Increase fiber intake.

3. Increase exercise and sunshine.
A daily walk in the sunshine can take care of both!

For getting a jump on preventing diabetes, here are the tests that are most helpful:

1. Fasting blood sugar and HbA1C
(glycosylated hemoglobin).
The latter screens for diabetes, measuring average blood sugar over the past few months.

2. Vitamin D levels.
Low vitamin D contributes to increased diabetes risk. Instead of checking vitamin D levels, be sure to take a multivitamin that contains 400–1,000 units of vitamin D. For overall health, look for a good multivitamin containing key nutrients (e.g., magnesium and many others) needed to maintain healthy blood sugar levels.

3. Testosterone levels.
These significantly increase diabetes risk if they are on the high side in women or too low in men. In men, consider treating with bioidentical testosterone cream or pellets if the testosterone level is under 450 ng/dL and/or they have symptoms of low libido or erectile dysfunction, especially if there are associated signs of metabolic syndrome (high cholesterol, prediabetes, and hypertension).

Thanks, or no thanks to medical "advances," right now, Americans are living long, unhealthy lives.

Yet we have choices. We always have choices. Diabetes—and all of the so-called "diseases of aging" are *totally optional.*

This is so important, we'll repeat it:

Diabetes—and all of the so-called "diseases of aging" are *totally optional.*

In the coming chapters, we'll tell you why and how.

CHAPTER 2
What is Diabetes?

Diabetes is a terrible disease on its own and because it spawns other deadly diseases.

Let's start with a little background. There are two types of diabetes, but we'll be focusing on only one—Type 2—for this book:

Type 1 diabetes is an autoimmune disease caused by the body's inability to produce insulin. It is usually diagnosed in children and young adults. People with Type 1 diabetes are insulin *deficient*. They are dependent on insulin for their entire lives and should absolutely use this treatment, although a healthy diet and exercise are also critical for them in order to enjoy long and healthy lives. According to the Juvenile Diabetes Research Foundation, about 40,000 children and young adults are diagnosed with Type 1 diabetes each year.

Type 2 diabetes results from insulin resistance, meaning the pancreas is producing sufficient (and often *excessive*) insulin. The problem is that for a variety of reasons, the body cannot use that insulin to turn the glucose in food into energy, a condition called insulin resistance. We'll be talking a lot more about insulin resistance in a couple of pages. Type 2 diabetes is a disease of long-term high blood sugar that impairs circulation and promotes inflammation that can result in a wide variety of problems, including heart disease, blindness, kidney failure, nerve damage and poor wound healing.

Type 2 diabetes is a lifestyle disease. Almost all people with the disease are overweight, inactive, and have a diet high in sugar and processed foods. It is an illness of Western civilization.

From Dr. Teitelbaum: *We said diabetes is reversible and I know this is true based on my extensive experience with my patients. Most of the answers are what you might expect: right diet and right exercise, and also a combination of balancing hormones and supplements that can have dramatic and impressive effects.*

At the top of my list of simple supplements is Hintonia latiflora, *from a tree that grows in the Sonoran Desert that is widely used in Mexico for diabetes and digestive complaints. But, Hintonia is far from a folk remedy. Sixty years of rigidly conducted scientific research in Germany shows that it is a very effective medicine. We'll delve more deeply into this miraculous herb in Chapter 6.*

But first, let's look a little further into diabetes, its causes and the ways we can prevent diabetes from gaining a foothold in your body and in your life. As you will see, diabetes is a life-altering disease that you really want to avoid or get rid of.

INSULIN RESISTANCE (IR)

A few paragraphs back, we mentioned that insulin resistance goes hand-in-hand with Type 2 diabetes. We won't burden you with an excessive amount of scientific gobbledygook, but let us give you some simple information that will help you understand what happens when your body can't adequately process the carbohydrates in your diet.

Your pancreas makes a hormone called insulin that plays a key part in using food—especially carbohydrates, for energy. Insulin plays a major role in metabolism—the way the body uses digested food for energy. The digestive tract breaks down carbohydrates—sugars and starches found in many foods—into glucose. Glucose is a form of sugar that enters the bloodstream. With the help of insulin, cells throughout the body absorb glucose and use it for energy.

An aside: We'll be using the terms "sugars" interchangeably with "glucose." Please understand that we're not just talking about table sugar when we use those words. All simple carbs convert quickly to glucose—whether they are sugary soft drinks, highly processed white flours or white rice. When we mention sugars, we mean all simple carbs.

WHAT DOES *INSULIN RESISTANCE* MEAN?

The more food you eat, the more insulin your body needs to produce. When blood glucose levels rise after a meal, the pancreas releases insulin to direct those sugars into the proper cells to be used for fuel. Insulin helps all of our body's cells absorb glucose from the bloodstream to be burned for energy, lowering blood glucose levels. It also stimulates the liver and muscle tissue to store excess glucose. The stored form of glucose is called glycogen. Insulin also lowers blood glucose levels by reducing glucose production in the liver.

When this system is not working properly, these calories get directed to your fat cells instead, causing massive weight gain that is hard to lose until you get the system working again.

In addition, high-sugar and simple-carbohydrate foods cause inflammation, and the body's own inflammatory reaction can further impair the ability of insulin to do its job, so the cells become starved for energy.

Insulin acts like a key to open cells to receive energy-producing glucose from the bloodstream. With insulin resistance, the cells don't open up to glucose, because they are deaf to the insulin.

If you are insulin resistant, your pancreas has to work overtime all the time to produce enough insulin to balance the carbohydrates in your diet. Eventually, the pancreas becomes overwhelmed by a high-sugar and high-carbohydrate diet.

When insulin can't do its job, and get glucose into the cells for energy, the cells become starved for energy. How ironic that a disease usually associated with overeating actually causes cells to starve!

Insulin resistance is a warning sign of diabetes, and it dramatically increases your chances of developing full-blown diabetes. Warning signs include high blood pressure, elevated cholesterol and abdominal weight gain (called a "spare tire"). The good news: It's not difficult to prevent, control or even reverse diabetes and its complications.

How can you tell if you are insulin resistant? Your doctor should occasionally order regular fasting blood glucose levels. If your fasting blood sugar is over 100 mg/dl, you have elevated blood sugar. We also consider a fasting insulin over 10 mIU/l to suggest insulin resistance. No need to panic! Keep reading. There's lots you can do.

Your doctor may also order a blood test called an HbA1C or blood glycosylated hemoglobin test. This is a much more definitive test because it averages your blood sugars over the past two to three months. If you ate that piece of birthday cake last night, it might raise your fasting blood sugar test results, but if you are metabolizing carbohydrates in a normal way, it would have little, if any, effect on your averages for the past three months. For people without diabetes, your HbA1C level should be 5.7 or lower. For people with diabetes who are aiming for tight control, your HbA1C level should be 7.0 or less. For people with Type 2 diabetes, an HbA1C of 7.0 or lower substantially reduces the risk for long-term problems.

WHAT CAUSES INSULIN RESISTANCE?

The most common cause of insulin resistance is metabolic syndrome, a deadly cluster of factors that also include obesity, especially around the waist, high blood pressure and elevated cholesterol and triglycerides (blood fats). (More about this in Chapter 3.)

Other factors associated with insulin resistance are:

- Obesity (without metabolic syndrome)
- Stress
- Pregnancy
- An infection or severe illness
- Steroid use
- Aging
- Insomnia and sleep apnea
- Smoking
- Fatty liver
- Acanthosis nigricans (darkening and thickening of skin)
- Polycystic ovary syndrome
- Reproductive abnormalities in women
- Ethnic origins, especially Latino, African-American, Native American or Asian

WHAT ARE THE COMPLICATONS OF DIABETES?

Long-term high blood sugar can cause a wide range of problems, including inflammation of the arteries and nerves, the source of most of the complications of diabetes.

Cardiovascular disease is the most common complication of diabetes. Many doctors treat people with newly diagnosed diabetes as if they have already had a heart attack, because the risk is so high. Because of the inflammation caused by long-term elevated blood sugar, people with diabetes have a high risk of heart attacks and strokes. Left untreated, blood vessel disease can also result in amputations.

Nerve damage, also called neuropathy is the result of nerve cells getting starved for energy, as well as inflammatory damage to the tiny capillaries that feed nerves, especially in the legs and feet, causing numbness, tingling and pain.

Poor wound healing is closely linked to neuropathy with the additional risk of slow healing wounds, fungal or bacterial infections. Left untreated, unhealed wounds can require amputation, so these should be addressed quickly.

Kidney damage or nephropathy occurs when the tiny blood vessels that feed the kidney begin to fail. Severe kidney damage requires dialysis or even a kidney transplant.

Eye damage (retinopathy) happens when the blood vessels that feed the retina of the eye are damaged due to chronically elevated blood sugars. Diabetes-related retinopathy is a primary cause of blindness. People with diabetes are also at higher risk of glaucoma and cataracts.

Alzheimer's disease is often called "diabetes of the brain," and even "Type 3 diabetes" for good reason. In Alzheimer's, the brain cells have difficulty taking up sugar. Meanwhile, the poorer your blood sugar control, the higher the risk of dementia, often because of mini-strokes.

As we've said before, diabetes and all of these side effects are *totally optional.* Remember: You are in charge!

CHAPTER 3
What is Metabolic Syndrome?

Put simply, metabolic syndrome is a basket of health conditions that add up to a greatly increased risk for diabetes and heart disease.

It's not a pretty picture. But again, as we've said in the past two chapters, the fact that diabetes and metabolic syndrome were once very rare shows that you have control over both. You can definitely prevent and reverse diabetes.

So the good news? A diagnosis of diabetes is not set in stone. It simply lets you know that your body wants you to take certain steps to promote health.

Three million new cases of metabolic syndrome are diagnosed in the U.S. each year and a shocking estimated 32% of Americans have the condition. Yet, most of the people who have metabolic syndrome, also sometimes called Syndrome X, don't even know it. There are few, if any, symptoms in the early stages, and the greatest indicator is a very visible one: abdominal obesity.

Here's the basket of the **Big Five** problems that lead to bigger problems:

1. Obesity

Of special significance is abdominal obesity—you know, that beer belly? For men, a waist circumference of 40 inches or more is an indicator of dangerous abdominal obesity and for women, a waist circumference of 35 inches or more is a warning sign. With more than two-thirds of American adults being overweight and one-third of us obese, this is a national epidemic that we must address. Read on, and we'll help you learn what to do.

Avoid Abdominal Obesity

- For men, a waist measurement of 40 inches or more
- For women, a waist measurement of 35 inches or more

2. High blood pressure

High blood pressure, also known as hypertension, is also distressingly common in the U.S., with one in three adults, 75 million of us, having this hidden time bomb. In today's stressful world, those numbers aren't really surprising, but they are worrisome. And, according to the Centers for Disease Control and Prevention, only a bit more than half of the people with high blood pressure have their numbers under optimal control. Yet, high blood pressure contributes to 1,100 deaths a day, says the CDC. It's definitely a problem! Your target blood pressure should be below 130/80. If it's higher than that in people with diabetes, elevated blood pressure is in itself a health risk and an important sign of metabolic syndrome.

3. High blood sugar

This means you have impaired sugar metabolism, and quite likely you have insulin resistance, as explained in Chapter 2. The simplest test is the finger prick using a blood glucose monitor. If your fasting blood sugar is over 100 mg/dL, you are at risk. It's best to check a glycosylated hemoglobin (HbA1C) and make sure it is 5.7 or less.

4. High cholesterol

High cholesterol is mostly one of those medical myths we'll discuss in an upcoming chapter. Moderately elevated cholesterol is not an especially important risk factor for causing heart disease or metabolic syndrome. It is not the main cause of the damage. Rather, it is like smoke from a fire.

Today's medical trend is to treat cholesterol levels with pharmaceuticals to make them so low they become dangerous. Although these drugs are very profitable for the drug companies, they really don't do much to help most people, unless they already have known heart disease. We could write an entire book on this subject. More on that in a couple of pages. What's more important is the level of HDL or "good" cholesterol. Women's levels should be over 50 mg/dL and men's over 40.

5. High blood fats

Blood fats, also known as triglycerides, store fat your body can use for energy. They're the end product of digesting and breaking down fats in food. If you eat more calories than you burn, those triglycerides find places to live—like on your hips and thighs. A healthy target for fasting triglycerides is 150 mg/dL or less.

As we said earlier, other than the visual sign of abdominal obesity, none of these risk factors for metabolic syndrome have noticeable symptoms. But if you're really fine-tuned, you may notice a few tiny things that can trigger that red warning light in your brain:

Fatigue, brain fog, thirst, frequent urination and darkening of skin in the neck, armpits, and groin can all be warning signs that one or more of the Big Five could be creeping up on you. Even simpler, just see your doctor and have a few simple and inexpensive blood tests. Then you'll know for sure.

THE BIG FIVE WARNING SIGNS FOR METABOLIC SYNDROME

1. **Abdominal Fat:** Waist circumference of over 40-inches for men, over 35 inches for women

2. **High Blood Pressure:** Over 130/80
3. **High Fasting Blood Sugar**: Over 100 mg/dL (or HbA1C over 5.7)
4. **High Cholesterol:** Total cholesterol over 250 mg/dL. HDL ""good" cholesterol should be over 40 for men or over 50 for women.
5. **High Triglycerides**: Over 150 mg/dL (fasting)

DEALING WITH THE BIG FIVE

First, let us make it clear: Having one or two or even all of the Big Five does not mean that you have irreversible metabolic syndrome or that diabetes and heart disease are the inevitable outcome.

Remember we said you're in control? You are. We mean it.

Let's go back over the Big Five and look at a few things you can do to reverse your situation and be healthier in the long run. We guarantee you, none of these are onerous. You don't have to turn your life upside down and subsist on grass and birdseed to be healthy and to beat metabolic syndrome. In fact, pleasure is a good thing. For example, chocolate, coffee, salt, and tea are all healthy for most people!

BIG BONUS FOR THE BIG FIVE

Before we get started on solutions, we're going to give you the Big Bonus—the simplest way to address *all* of the Big Five:

Get moving! It's as simple as that. Walking just 30 minutes five days a week has been shown to reduce abdominal fat, lower blood sugar, lower blood pressure, lower cholesterol, and drop triglycerides. It's easy—anybody can do it. You can do it virtually anywhere and all you need is a good pair of shoes. You don't have to get sweaty and you don't even have to do the entire 30 minutes at once. Ten-minute increments are easy to fit into the busiest schedule. Sunshine makes your walk even more effective, since low vitamin D (the sunshine vitamin) is associated with diabetes.

Who could ask for more?

1. Obesity/Abdominal Fat

Lots of research shows that abdominal fat is the most dangerous kind because it builds up around your internal organs. That fat makes particular kinds of toxins, including inflammatory cytokines that increase the risk of insulin resistance and heart disease. How to get rid of abdominal fat? The easy answer: Get moving, get more sunshine, eat less sugar and processed food and eat more fiber.

2. High Blood Pressure

The easiest answer is stress relief. What chills you out? Of course, I'm advocating walking, but how about listening to music, taking a long bubbly bath or curling up with a favorite cup of tea? Also, ditch the junk food and keep your caffeine and alcohol to three servings of each or less daily. Oh, and feel free to add up to an ounce of dark chocolate a day. Studies show that small amounts (under an ounce a day) can lower blood pressure by 3 or 4 points. Uh, no, that doesn't mean that five ounces will lower blood pressure by 20 points. Nice try!

Especially important? Increase potassium intake with foods such as tomato juice, coconut water, avocados and bananas. These can lower blood pressure 5–10 mm. Strictly limiting salt intake is less important, only lowering average blood pressure by 3 mm. Perhaps the new expression should be "A banana a day keeps the doctor away."

3. High Fasting Blood Sugar

This one is pretty much a no-brainer: lower the amounts of sugar and simple carbs in your diet. Start by cutting out sodas and fruit juices (although whole fruits are fine). Avoid sweets (an occasional treat is fine) and increase the fiber in your diet. Fiber slows digestion and keeps blood sugar levels balanced. The best sources of fiber include whole grains, legumes (dried beans), fruits and vegetables.

4. High Cholesterol

First, don't worry about eggs. Studies show that even eating six eggs a day (who wants to do that?) has no effect on blood cholesterol levels. Eat whole grain oatmeal for breakfast, season with garlic and snack on a handful of mono-unsaturated tree nuts (walnuts, almond, pecans) daily. Here's a little bit of interesting science: Studies show eating oatmeal and garlic (not necessarily together!) can lower cholesterol nearly as much at prescription statin drugs without the negative side effects. And have we mentioned chocolate? Small amounts each day have been associated with a 57% lower risk of heart attack death. As cholesterol medications only lower heart attack death about 5% in those who don't have angina or a history of heart attack, this makes a small square of chocolate each day about 10 times as beneficial as cholesterol.

See, we told you it wouldn't be hard!

5. High Triglycerides

The guidelines for lowering cholesterol stand as well for lowering triglycerides.

You may have noticed that increased dietary fiber is almost a universal way to improve risks for metabolic syndrome and improve your health. Fruits and vegetables are probably the best sources of fiber, but whole grains and legumes can be important sources of fiber and protein.

CHAPTER 4
It's a Reversible Lifestyle Disease

When we said that diabetes is reversible, we weren't exaggerating. As we told you earlier, diabetes used to be very rare. Reversing the problem requires some changes, and those changes are part of your lifestyle that you can control.

So sometimes simple lifestyle choices can change your life. In some cases, it can banish diabetes completely, even if you've had the disease for years.

Consider this: Extensive research shows that bariatric surgery (stomach stapling or gastric bypass) can reverse diabetes in as little as three weeks. How does this work? By limiting the amount of food a person can eat, weight goes down. A review of dozens of scientific studies showed that 78.1% of patients who have the surgery no longer have diabetes and 86.6% showed improvement in their blood sugar control by losing an average of 84.7 pounds.

Before we go any farther, let us say unequivocally that you don't need drastic measures like bariatric surgery. And you don't have to lose 85 pounds. Our point here is that you can get the excellent results by making some fairly easy—and often fun—lifestyle changes.

Here's a critical clue:

The Standard American Diet (SAD), full of processed foods, sugar and harmful fats, is killing us. The acronym "SAD" is an appropriate one. Our heavily processed diet is at the heart of the obesity and diabetes epidemic. You can't separate them.

But hundreds of years ago, before diabetes was a problem, people really savored their food and their diet. They ate and enjoyed life with gusto. And so can you.

Type 2 diabetes and overweight are so closely related that some experts call the problem "diabesity." One theory about the connection: Insulin resistance can be triggered by problems with our mitochondrial energy furnaces. When these organelles that convert food to energy for the cells to use stop working properly, the production of health-destroying free radicals (oxidants) increases, so healthy antioxidants can be very helpful.

So insulin resistance is not only caused by being overweight, but may be the reason that you are overweight. And it all traces back to our diet.

We know, every doctor you've seen has told you that you have to shed a few pounds. Your doc may even be telling you that while stealthily adjusting a white coat to cover a paunch. We also know that it's easier said than done.

Have heart. It's easier than you think.

Here's the drill:

Eat fewer processed foods and sugar, more healthy fats and proteins, and walk a few more miles each week.

There's lots of good research that proves that these simple lifestyle changes work.

One of the biggest studies took place more than 15 years ago. The Diabetes Prevention Program, conducted by the National Institute of Diabetes and Digestive and Kidney Diseases, divided more than 3,000 overweight people with prediabetes in 27 centers into one of three programs for three years:

1. A lifestyle program that focused on weight loss through fat and calorie reduction (their target was to lose 7% of their body weight) and increased exercise (150 minutes a week).
2. A group that took 850 mg of metformin, a pharmaceutical for diabetes twice daily.
3. A group that was given a placebo pill.

Both the metformin group and the placebo group were given information about diet and exercise, but no counseling or follow-up.

Researchers were tremendously excited by the results: Participants in the lifestyle group reduced their risk of developing full-blown Type 2 diabetes by an impressive 58% and people over 60 had an even better result—a 71% reduced risk of diabetes. The metformin group reduced the risk of developing diabetes by 31% and the placebo group by just 11%.

This is proof positive that we can take charge of our lives and prevent diabetes (and heart disease and strokes and more) without reliance on pharmaceuticals with myriad side effects.

Stay with us. It's easy:

YOUR DIABETES PREVENTION EATING PLAN

1. Eat more fiber

A diet rich in fresh vegetables, a moderate amount of fruit (no fruit juices though), whole grains and legumes (dried beans) are filling and friendly to your weight.

2. Limit your intake of fatty foods

Limit fried foods and junk foods that increase oxidative stress in your mitochondrial energy furnaces. Look at your portion sizes. A proper portion of meat would be about the size of your hand. If you want a snack, grab some veggies, a piece of fruit or whole grain crackers dipped in hummus.

3. Limit sugar

Dr. Teitelbaum admits he has a sweet tooth, but we all know that we can't overindulge it without paying a price, including opening ourselves to Type 2 diabetes. Avoid sodas completely. They are loaded with sugar. Stevia is a healthier sugar substitute. It also sweetens iced tea or lemonade very nicely. And you can even bake with it and indulge your sweet tooth safely. Although any sweet drink can trigger some insulin release (likely just from the sweet taste buds on your tongue being stimulated), regular sodas seem to do so more than diet sodas.

4. Drink more water

Water fills you up. You should drink at least ½ ounce of water for every pound you weigh, so if you weigh 150 pounds, drink at least 75 ounces of water a day, more if it's hot or you are exercising.

YOUR DIABETES PREVENTION EXERCISE PLAN

1. This is simple: **Intentionally exercise 150 minutes a week.** That's not at all difficult. It's only 21.42 minutes a day. Plus, you don't have to do it all in one session. A ten-minute walk at lunchtime and another after dinner or a quick after-work game of tennis or a Zumba® class—they all count. Many people

like to wear fitness bands or pedometers and aim for 10,000 steps a day (about 5 miles). You'd be surprised how easy it is.

2. **What kind of exercise should you do?** That answer is simple, too: Do what you love. It will come easily and you will stick to it. If you love walking in the woods but you'd rather have a root canal than play tennis, there's your answer. Also, schedule a time into your routine to exercise and do it with a friend (or your dog). This way, you are much more likely to show up and not make excuses!

A final word on weight control to prevent diabetes: No matter how much excess weight you carry, remember that the Diabetes Prevention Program showed profound results for people who had a target of just 7% of body weight lost in three years. If you weigh 200 pounds, that's just 21 pounds. You can do that. Research has shown that weight loss can reverse as many as 85% of cases of diabetes.

A mixed metaphor to carry with you: How do you eat an elephant? One bite at a time. If you drop just half a pound a week, that's 26 pounds a year.

Before we end this chapter, we'd like to share with you a few common medical myths that you will be thrilled to find have been busted—not just as they apply to Type 2 diabetes, but to your overall health. You'll see how deeply committed we are to simplicity and loving life's pleasures. Enjoy!

11 COMMON MEDICAL MYTHS THAT YOU WILL BE THRILLED HAVE BEEN BUSTED

1. Men should undergo a **PSA screening test** annually to catch prostate cancer early. BUSTED! Screening tests for prostate cancer have been shown to have no effect on saving or prolonging lives, but do result in very toxic, frightening and expensive treatments (but men died at the same age whether or not they did the test).

2. Women should have **mammograms** every year after 40: BUSTED! The U.S. Preventive Services Task Force changed mammogram recommendations from yearly after age 40 to every other year ages 50–74, unless a woman is at high risk for breast cancer. Due to high "false positives" with increasing numbers of mammograms over the year, many women are opting for thermograms instead.

3. Early **screening for osteoporosis** saves lives if you are limited to standard treatment. BUSTED! Routine screening with DEXA scans is no longer recommended till age 65 unless a person is high risk. Meanwhile, the major osteoporosis medications were shown to cause as much fracture risk as they prevented after five years' use. On the other hand, a low-cost mineral called strontium is being shown in long-term placebo-controlled studies to be safe and VERY effective, making the DEXA screening again worthwhile.

4. Salt restriction is important for high blood pressure. BUSTED! Severe restriction only drops BP three points. Yet another study in the *Journal of the American Medical Association* shows a low-salt diet results in four times the death rate from heart disease. Two other large studies show salt restriction to the government recommendations markedly increases likelihood of dying younger. Eat unrefined sea salt—preferably the ones that are pink or gray because they are packed with essential minerals. We like Himalayan sea salt. Instead, limit the amount of salt in processed foods.

5. Avoid eggs. BUSTED AGAIN! In a meta-analysis of over 250,000 people, "This meta-analysis identified no significant association between egg consumption and risk of coronary heart disease or stroke. Higher intake of eggs (up to one egg per day) was not associated with risk of coronary heart disease or stroke." Earlier studies showed that even six eggs a day had minimal to no effects on cholesterol levels.

6. Avoid coffee and tea. BUSTED! These are actually healthy. No, this isn't Starbucks' PR firm talking to you. It's the take-home message from a study conducted by researchers at the National Cancer

Institute. They analyzed 13 years of health data from more than 400,000 people and found that people who drank 3–4 cups of coffee a day reduced their risk of early death by 12–13% compared to folks who didn't drink coffee. Looking at specific health problems, the researchers found coffee drinking was linked to fewer deaths from diabetes, heart disease, respiratory disease, stroke, injuries, accidents and infections. Like tea, coffee is plant-based and chock full of antioxidants and other wonderful nutrients. (I would keep it to 1–2 cups a day, and switch to decaf if having more.) Meanwhile, tea lowers heart attack and Alzheimer's risk and even lowers cholesterol, and green tea can be helpful in a weight-loss program.

7. Chocolate is bad for you. HAPPILY BUSTED! Chocolate is more effective than cholesterol medications at decreasing heart disease. Researchers from the University of Cambridge analyzed seven studies on chocolate and heart health involving more than 114,000 people. Compared to those who ate the *least* chocolate, those who ate the most had a 37% reduced rate of any type of cardiovascular disease (angina, heart attack, heart failure), a 57% lower risk of heart attack death and a 29% reduced risk of stroke. The chocolate lovers also had a 35% lower risk of developing diabetes and a 50% lower risk of dying from heart disease. To put that finding in perspective, the cholesterol-lowering statin drugs decrease the initial risk of getting heart disease (called primary prevention) by only 2 to 10%. That means chocolate is more than 10 times more powerful than statins in protecting your heart! (Not to mention a whole lot tastier!) But more is not better, because this is not a low-calorie food. So go for quality not quantity as an occasional treat.

8. Avoid Sunshine. VERY BUSTED! Avoiding sunshine is deadly. For starters, inadequate vitamin D is associated with a significantly increased risk of diabetes. It is estimated that the current advice to avoid sunshine, our main source of vitamin D, had contributed to hundreds of thousands of unnecessary deaths from many types of cancer, diabetes, and autoimmune disease. The proper advice? Avoid sunburn, not sunshine! Vitamin D deficiency is becoming alarmingly common since the misguided medical advice to avoid sunshine (which is the source of over 90% of our vitamin D) and wear sunscreen all the time. Vitamin D is not only a vitamin, but also an important hormone, with deficiencies causing widespread health problems. In addition to the above, therapy with vitamin D can also improve lung function and help people with asthma, while also decreasing the risk of heart disease, hypertension, and stroke. For those with decreased bone density, 2,000–4,000 units a day are best. Otherwise, 1,000–2,000 units a day is optimal.

Most important, remember to go for walks and get your sunshine, which is good for you.

9. Calcium supplements prevent osteoporosis. ANOTHER MYTH BUSTED Calcium supplements have minimal, if any, benefit, but in men may increase heart attack risk by a whopping 20–47%. Because of this, when giving calcium antacids, it is critical that they also contain magnesium, vitamin K and vitamin D to avoid this problem.

10. Arthritis meds are safe. NOT BY A LONG SHOT! These medications, called NSAIDs, include medications in the ibuprofen family. They kill over 30,000 Americans a year unnecessarily, 16,500 of them from bleeding ulcers and a 40% increased risk of heart attack and stroke.

Why do we say these deaths are preventable? Because multiple studies have shown natural options to be as or more effective in head on double-blinded, controlled studies. These include a special highly bioavailable form of curcumin (which is being associated with a $^{2}/_{3}$ lower risk of Alzheimer's and a strong anticancer effect), glucosamine (associated with a 17% lower risk of dying during one large study), boswellia (frankincense), chondroitin and others. In addition to having "side benefits" instead of side effects (like killing you), these natural options are much less expensive.

The medications have the benefit of starting to work quicker though. The good news? The natural options can be added to the medications, and both can often be stopped once the arthritis pain is gone for three months.

Dr. Teitelbaum's first "go to" supplement for people with pain or arthritis is curcumin. In head-to-head studies, a unique form of curcumin blended with turmeric essential oil was more effective than prescription drugs at relieving pain.

11. YOUR DOCTOR KNOWS EVERYTHING THAT CAN HELP YOU. This is the most important health myth ever. **BUSTED! BUSTED! BUSTED!** In truth, medicine only offers less than 25% of what can help. Modern medicine's greatest strength is in acute, life threatening conditions, such as heart attacks or traumatic injuries. Integrative medicine (sometimes called functional medicine and what we like to call Comprehensive Medicine, a term coined by the late and great Dr. Hugh Riordan) offers the rest of the healing arts toolkit, e.g., for pain, fatigue, and chronic health conditions such as arthritis, diabetes and heart failure. So if your doctor says, "I can't help you," just say, "Thank you for being honest." Then, instead of going home to die or suffer, simply go to an integrative medicine practitioner who can help you!

CHAPTER 5
Conventional Treatment for Diabetes: Down the Rabbit Hole

Conventional treatments for diabetes sometimes cause more harm than good.

So, you went to the doctor and after some routine tests, he tells you that your fasting blood sugar is high. Too high. It's not prediabetes, it's the real Magilla: Type 2 diabetes.

If you feel like you're Alice falling down the rabbit hole with such a dire diagnosis, it doesn't help that conventional doctors tend to pile on until you're scared, confused, and confounded.

You fall into a funk. You'll never be able to eat another piece of guilt-free birthday cake or chow down on fried dough at your town's fall festival.

Too much of these things is not healthy for anyone, and having diabetes means you need to be conscious of what you eat, but it doesn't mean a life of deprivation.

DIABETES DRUGS

Diabetes is almost always treated with prescription drugs. Most of these drugs can lead to the rabbit hole we warned you about. None is perfect, and almost all have serious side effects. That said, please do not ever discontinue a medicine, especially a diabetes medicine, without consulting your doctor.

Until then, isn't it wonderful there is a better way?

Biguanides: The most commonly used diabetes medications belong to a group called biguanides that decrease the amount of sugar the liver makes while also decreasing the amount of sugar absorbed by the intestines, making the body more sensitive to insulin and helping muscles absorb glucose.

Metformin is the most common of the biguanides. It is prescribed under the brand names Glucophage, Metformin Hydrochloride ER, Glumetza, Riomet, Fortamet and combined with other medication in several drugs.

Biguanides can have uncomfortable side effects, but they are generally not life threatening. If you must take a diabetes drug, metformin is the safest until you can get your sugars under control with natural supplements and lifestyle changes.

The most serious side effect of metformin is that it will cause B12 deficiency. So please be sure to take a multivitamin that contains a high level of vitamin B12.

Dr. Teitelbaum doesn't use the other drugs listed below because historically other diabetes medications are found to cause more harm than benefit in the long term. He much prefers controlling diabetes naturally. But here are some other common diabetes meds.

Sulfonylureas: This is among the oldest diabetes drugs used today which works by stimulating the pancreas to produce more insulin. These drugs include: glimepride (Amaryl), glimepride pioglitzazone (Duetact), glimepride-rospglitazone (Avandaryl), glipezide (Glucotrol), toilbutamide (Orinase and Tol-Tab) and several more.

Side effects of these drugs include weight gain, hunger, hypoglycemia (low blood sugar) with its symptoms, including dizziness, sweating, confusion and nervousness, upset stomach and skin irritation.

Thiazolidinediones (also called TZDs or glitazones) These work by decreasing glucose in the liver. They help fat cells use insulin more effectively. They include rosiglitazone (Avandia), rosiglitazone-metformin (Amaryl M), rosiglitazone-glimepride (Avandaryl), pioglitazone (Actos), and several others.

Side effects of these drugs are significant. They can cause heart disease, most commonly congestive heart failure, in people with Type 2 diabetes who are already at high risk for heart disease and may have already experienced it. Other side effects include increased

LDL (bad) cholesterol, increase risk of bone fracture, weight gain, and edema (water retention).

Insulin is necessary for anyone with Type 1 diabetes. It's a very different story for Type 2 diabetes, however. Deteriorating glucose control over time sometimes prompts physicians to prescribe insulin for people who have Type 2 diabetes, with higher levels needed as time passes. This is another sign that diabetes itself causes the weight gain, worsening the blood sugar control over time—unless you take matters into your own hands!

Today's insulin pharmacopoeia offers five basic types of insulin. All are injectable.

- Short-acting (old-style insulin): sold under the brand names Humalin and Novolin
- Rapid acting: Novolog, FlexPen, Apidra, Humalog
- Intermediate acting: Humulin N, Novolin N
- Long-acting: Tresiba, Levemir, Lantus, Toujeo
- Combination: Novolog Mix, Humalog Mix, Ryuzodeg

Side effects: The most common side effect of all types of insulin is hypoglycemia or low blood sugar. Since most of us eat varied types of food and are rarely on a strict eating schedule, dosage needs may vary. It's fairly easy to miscalculate the correct dosage, thereby causing hypoglycemia. Many people with Type 2 diabetes have difficulty recognizing the symptoms of hypoglycemia, which can include dizziness, sweating, fast heartbeat, blurry vision, and hunger.

On the other hand, if blood sugars go too high, the symptoms are much more difficult to recognize. They can include extreme thirst, frequent urination, rapid breathing, flushing, fruity smelling breath, and confusion.

If blood sugars drop too low or rise too high, they can result in a diabetic coma, which is life threatening.

The biggest problem? In adult diabetics, treating with insulin often causes massive weight gain. This worsens insulin resistance and the diabetes. Basically, it is a diabetes "loan shark."

The bottom line: We prefer natural treatments over prescription medications for Type 2 diabetes. Be an ambassador for healthy healthcare. Find healthcare professionals who will work with you to treat Type 2 diabetes with achievable lifestyle changes and consider using Hintonia to prevent deteriorating blood sugar control and the need for more medications.

CHAPTER 6
Hintonia: The Herbal Answer to Type 2 Diabetes, Prediabetes, and Metabolic Syndrome

You can stop diabetes without medications.

Let us repeat that: You can stop diabetes without medications.

High blood sugar, Type 2 diabetes and metabolic syndrome are *not* inevitable. A diagnosis of Type 2 diabetes is *not* a life sentence.

Whatever the dire statistics may tell you (and your doctor), you can stabilize, reverse and normalize your blood sugar levels with the lifestyle changes we talked about in Chapter 4, with the help of an amazing herbal extract!

Clinical research has now confirmed what the indigenous people of Mexico have known for centuries: *Hintonia latiflora* is effective for, and often reverses mild to moderate Type 2 diabetes!

Found in marketplaces in Mexico and Central America, this miracle botanical is an extract of the bark of a shrubby tree that grows in the Sonoran Desert.

Its medicinal power comes from the extreme climate changes the tree experiences in its desert home.

The desert's scorching heat and torrential rainfalls stress the *Hintonia latiflora* tree and provide the keys to a powerful defense mechanism inherent in the plant and an essential part of its medicinal value. The natural environmental stresses to the tree enhance its ability to survive and thrive in such a harsh environment and are key to Hintonia's traditional use to treat Type 2 diabetes and gastrointestinal problems.

But Hintonia is much more than a folk remedy. It's been studied in detail for its ability to reverse high blood sugars for over 60 years.

The earliest work showed that Hintonia extract is often as effective in lowering blood sugar as insulin and even more effective in some cases. But Hintonia results in "side benefits" instead of side effects. That early research was done even before the days of oral diabetes medications.

Since then, there have been over a dozen studies showing how powerfully effective Hintonia is!

Today's widespread availability of oral diabetes medications has decreased the number of adult diabetics taking long-term insulin. However, as we learned in Chapter 5, those diabetes medications carry serious side effects with them. Furthermore, why would you want your condition to deteriorate, requiring progressively more potent medications with increasingly serious side effects? It sounds like it is definitely time for a better solution.

The good news? Hintonia to the rescue!

Plants and plant extracts are composed of complex molecules, usually with a variety of nutrients that are dependent on one another to act synergistically or to enhance each other.

Hintonia is no exception.

HOW DOES HINTONIA WORK?

First, it is a rich source of flavonoids, nutritional compounds found in colorful fruits and vegetables. Extensive research shows that flavonoids reduce insulin resistance and inflammation.

Flavonoids are great, but if all flavonoids prevented diabetes, you could eat a bunch of grapes or tomatoes or drink a lot of red wine and that would do the trick. Unfortunately, that's not the case. Hintonia stands alone in the gift of blood sugar control.

But more about that later in this chapter. Let's start by looking at the research on Hintonia and how it helps reverse diabetes.

Solid research shows that not only can Hintonia help control blood sugar and overcome insulin resistance, reducing your need for pharmaceuticals, it can also enhance the effectiveness of diabetes medications if your doctor and you decide that you need them.

In fact, in a study published in the German journal *Naturheilpraxis mit Naturalmedizin* (*Naturopathic Practice with Natural Medicine*) the dry concentrated bark extract of *Hintonia latiflora*—combined with additional nutrients—significantly lowered HbA1C values (average levels of blood sugar), fasting glucose levels (blood sugar before a meal) and postprandial (after eating) blood sugar levels.

Fasting and after meal blood glucose numbers, along with HbA1C levels, are important because they show how much sugar circulates through your system and how your body deals with it after meals. What the research showed was amazing! Fasting and post-meal blood sugars improved by an impressive 23% and 24% respectively with Hintonia. And glycosylated hemoglobin decreased by a remarkable average of 0.8 points! (about 11%). This means many people went from being diabetic to no longer being diabetic.

Impressively, by the end of the study, 39% of those using anti-diabetes drugs could reduce their medication levels. Some were able to stop their diabetes medications entirely.

But there is more good news. Hintonia not only lowers blood sugar and often reverses diabetes. It also eliminates many of the symptoms of diabetes.

One study factored in a mix of major diabetic symptoms. The scores improved an impressive 73%, from an average 4.8 points to 1.3 points at the end of the study. This is a massive change that can dramatically increase your quality of life and well-being.

Participants also saw improvements in blood pressure, lipids and liver values.

Other valuable studies of Hintonia show that compounds from its leaves may help stop gastrointestinal damage and gastric ulcers. Considering the gastrointestinal discomfort caused by some drugs used for Type 2 diabetes, this is yet another reason to consider adding *Hintonia latiflora* to a diabetes-fighting regimen.

STOP THE BLOOD SUGAR ROLLER COASTER

People with diabetes struggle with blood sugars that spike and plummet during the day and night. As this occurs, your energy, pain, and mental clarity may find themselves on a roller coaster as well.

One of Hintonia's greatest benefits is that it helps keep those sugars steady throughout the day and night, making life easier and contributing to better long-term glucose control.

Mexican researchers were finally able to isolate the unique way that it works: The plant is an inhibitor of alpha-glucosidase, an enzyme that releases sugar from foods, particularly carbohydrates. We all know that carbohydrates, especially simple carbs like sugar and foods made with white flour, are the bugaboo of people with Type 2 diabetes, so this news alone is a huge boon for people with the disease.

Coutareagenin, a polyphenol nutrient found in the bark extracts unique to Hintonia, appears to be responsible for many of its other blood-sugar-controlling benefits. For this reason, please seek out a Hintonia supplement standardized to contain at least 20 mg of coutareagenin polyphenols, taken two to three times daily.

The president of the International Diabetes Foundation was the lead author on another study that strongly recommended the use of this unique herb in treating and preventing Type 2 diabetes. Not only because of improved blood sugar control, but also because of its effectiveness in lowering cholesterol and other elements of metabolic syndrome that can lead to Type 2 diabetes.

Finally, in yet another clinical study, adult participants with Type 2 diabetes were provided with an extract of *Hintonia latiflora* combined with trace nutrients (vitamins B1, B6, B12, folic acid, chromium, zinc and vitamins C and E) for six months. These ingredients also help protect against oxidative damage to blood vessels, stop nerve damage and keep metabolism functioning the way that it should. But it is the Hintonia that is the heavy hitter.

WHERE DOES HINTONIA COME FROM?

The Hintonia bark is grown and harvested in the upper zones (highlands) and part of the Petén (jungle area) in Guatemala. The bush can be found as well in Mexico, El Salvador, Honduras and other countries in Central

America. There are even scientific reports in Spanish on this special herb written in the 1950s.

Hintonia is grown and harvested wild and also in specific fields where a technique called vegetative reproduction is used. Once one plant is harvested, parts of its root are taken and planted somewhere else, resulting in a new bush with exactly the same properties and content of polyphenols.

The bark containing the valuable polyphenols is peeled off by a worker. To protect the plant, however, only the upper layers are taken away, with the bark layers below remaining. This way they ensure that the Hintonia bush stays alive and healthy, and the bark, the lifeline where the nutrients, water, etc. are transported between the roots and crown of the bush continues to be intact. This *very careful and labor-intensive way* of harvesting is essential to protect these precious bushes and prevents overharvesting.

We highly recommend adding a clinically studied *Hintonia latiflora* product, to your daily regimen. Look for one that also contains B-vitamins, folic acid, chromium, zinc, and vitamins C and E.

CHAPTER 7
So What Can I Eat if I Have Type 2 Diabetes?

We've said it before, but it's worth saying it again: Having Type 2 diabetes does not mean you have to give up all of the sweet things in life. Not at all. But you do have to find a path of moderation. We're the first to admit that is difficult. Remember Dr, Teitelbaum told you about his sweet tooth? Well, it's still there, but he has learned over time how to indulge himself healthfully.

You can find the balance.

Here are a few tips that will get you on the right track:

Don't eat white. Fiber is found in fruits and vegetables. It's also plentiful in dried beans and whole grains. Let's look at some white foods—sugar, white rice, white bread, and white pasta. These are all simple carbohydrates and, like pure sugar, they are all digested quickly and cause blood sugar spikes while adding virtually no nutrients to your diet. With Type 2 diabetes, your glucose metabolism is impaired, so those simple carbohydrates contribute to blood sugar swings. But there's an easy solution: Go for whole grain breads, pastas and the occasional baked goods—in moderation, of course. Whole grains are fiber rich, meaning they are digested much more slowly than simple carbs, and they help you avoid blood sugar swings. Fiber is also filling, so you can eat less bulk and fewer calories and still feel satisfied.

Portion control. There's the rub. Yes, with diabetes you can eat much more than docs once told you, but you still need to be conscious of the quantity you eat. Since almost all people with Type 2 diabetes are overweight, getting your weight under control will help you get diabetes in hand, too. It's not your fault—there is no blame here. Remember the blood sugar roller coaster? It's well known that diabetes makes your body think it is starving, especially triggering cravings for sweets when your last sugar high starts to wear off. It's not just mind over matter. When you crave something sweet, reach for protein instead—unsweetened yogurt, a hard-boiled egg, a handful of pumpkin seeds, an occasional handful of nuts or some string cheese.

Just a rule of thumb (pun intended!): A serving of meat is approximately the size of the palm of your hand. A serving of raw veggies (think salad) is about the amount you can hold in two cupped hands. A small baked potato is about the size of a computer mouse, a cup of broccoli or carrots is about the size of a baseball, and a cup of mashed potatoes is about the size of a light bulb. You may want to measure carefully until you get the hang of it. Eating slowly, chewing well and avoiding distractions like TV during mealtimes will help you get through the initial idea that you want more.

Here is a simple trick that you will find very helpful. It takes 30 minutes for your stomach to get the signal to the brain that you are full. This is why when you eat until you feel full, you find yourself uncomfortably bloated a half hour later.

So begin with small portions, giving yourself permission to take seconds a half hour later. Most of the time, you'll find that you are full a half hour later and won't need to take more.

Ditch sugar and sweeteners. Yes, we love sweet stuff. We're hardwired to look for the sweetest, ripest, most nutritious fruits. We'll make a categorical statement here: Fat doesn't make you fat, sugar and simple carbs do.

If you have metabolic syndrome, prediabetes or Type 2 diabetes, the sugar has got to go. Our taste buds do recognize anything that tastes sweet and will stimulate some insulin in response. But they do not cause the rapid rise in blood sugar that eating sugar does. So although it is not a perfect solution, I do consider stevia to be acceptable. Saccharin (Sweet'n Low—the pink packet) is artificial, but not as toxic as aspartame (Nutrasweet, Equal, Sugar Twin). Sucralose (Splenda) may alter natural insulin production and have other negative side effects.

Aspartame has been linked to severe headaches and depression. Most interesting, aspartame has been strongly linked to increased extreme hunger, pretty much undoing any idea that it's a diet tool. Despite all this, we do consider diet sodas to be a much better choice than regular sodas, which have three quarters of a teaspoon of sugar per ounce (same as fruit juices by the way). So that 48-ounce "Big Burp" soda has a toxic 36 spoons of sugar!

Go for the good stuff: Stevia is sweet, natural and much healthier, and you can find stevia-sweetened sodas at your health food store and even supermarkets now. It will help feed your sweet tooth gently. Better yet, enjoy one or two fruits each day. An orange contains about two teaspoons of sugar, as opposed to 12 teaspoons of sugar for a 16-ounce orange juice. This way, you can satisfy your sweet tooth healthfully and add a ton of nutrients you won't get in soft drinks.

If you are going to have some candy, make it chocolate and keep it to less than an ounce a day. Go for the best tasting one you can and savor it. In moderation, chocolate is a health food, and eating about half an ounce a day is associated with a 50% lower risk of heart attack death. But it is high-calorie and has a fair bit of sugar (the darker the chocolate, the less sugar), so go for quality not quantity!

Consider Paleo or Ketogenic: Low carb diets can be helpful for people with diabetes. The Paleolithic and ketogenic diets are currently being followed by millions of people with a good success rate. This has been the answer for many people with Type 2 diabetes and has been shown to reduce dependence on anti-diabetes drugs, improve symptoms of metabolic syndrome, and even reverse the disease.

We haven't seen research on these diets combined with Hintonia, but it's a pretty good guess that they'd make a powerful diabetes-busting combo.

The Paleo diet focuses on foods that would have been available to our Paleolithic ancestors, 2.5 million to 10,000 years ago. It largely consists of lean meats, fish, fruits, vegetables, seeds and nuts, and minimizes consumption of dairy products and grains.

The ketogenic diet is high fat, moderate protein and low carbohydrate, forcing the body to burn fats rather than carbs for fuel. Much like the Paleo diet, the keto diet focuses on meats, fish and vegetables, but it also adds dairy and eggs, keeping carb consumption below 50 grams per day. More good news? Your cells can burn the ketones for fuel even if you are insulin resistant. So your cells can finally start to get the energy they need safely, and your hunger pains will start to disappear!

These diets provide sufficient daily fats and proteins—but very few carbs—which means the body's energy comes from using body fat and fats from the diet. Fats provide ketones, which are used for energy in the place of glucose. They also suppress your appetite. When you essentially "train" your body to stop using glucose as its primary source of energy, you help break the addiction to sugars and carbs and reduce your risk of diabetes.

For some people, following a diet this exacting can seem tough. We recommend working into it a little at a time, gradually getting yourself away from refined starches and sugars. We think you'll notice a positive difference that will make you want to continue on this course.

There are loads of books, websites and videos about both diets for those of you who are interested in giving them a try.

BETTER BLOOD SUGAR SHOPPING LIST

- Eggs
- Unprocessed meats: Beef, pork, lamb, chicken, turkey and duck
- Trout, salmon, cod, shrimp and tuna
- Vegetables including broccoli, cabbage, spinach, cauliflower, carrots, celery, peppers, cucumbers, sweet potatoes, and beets
- Natural, non-hydrolyzed fats, including butter, coconut oil, olive oil and avocado oil
- Nuts, including almonds, walnuts, macadamias, pecans and sunflower seeds
- Berries, including blueberries, raspberries, strawberries, and other fruits

SAMPLE DIET AND EXERCISE PLANS

From Dr. Teitelbaum:

Because I have been asked about the right diet and workout so many times, I have outlined a meal plan that goes into a bit more detail than the list above, but is more stringent, and an exercise program that is simple and effective, and included it in this book. I think you'll find that as you follow each to get control of your blood sugar, other benefits will follow; you'll lose unwanted weight, tone up your muscles, have more energy and improve your stamina.

To get you started, here's a sample menu for a day.

BREAKFAST

- 2–4 eggs any style cooked in butter, olive oil, coconut oil or lard
- $^{1}/_{2}$ grapefruit or other low GI (Glycemic Index) fruit
- 2–4 slices of bacon (no preservatives such as nitrates or nitrites)
- Cup of coffee or green tea with whole cream

Mid-Morning Snack

- $^{1}/_{4}$ cup raw almonds or walnuts

Or

- 1 boiled egg, 1 fruit choice

LUNCH

- Choice of animal protein
- Non-starchy vegetables seasoned with olive oil or butter and Celtic sea salt
- 1 piece fresh fruit—see suggestion in the snack list
- Unsweetened iced tea with lemon, coffee or green tea

Mid-Afternoon Snack

- 1 serving of cheese
- Small handful of walnuts

DINNER

- Unlimited salad (lettuce, tomatoes, cucumbers, avocado, peppers, mushrooms, etc. seasoned with olive oil and Celtic sea salt)
- Choice of animal protein
- Steamed broccoli, snow peas, asparagus, zucchini, etc. dressed with either butter or olive oil and Celtic sea salt

Dessert

- Small apple, pear, plum, peach, apricot or grapefruit

Bedtime Snack

- Small handful of nuts or seeds and 1 ounce cheese

Snacking

Yes, you can snack whenever you want on this type of diet! It's not required, and you may not even feel like snacking since the diet is so complete and satisfying.

- Chopped raw vegetables, raw cheese or nut butter
- Slices of cold meat such as turkey, chicken or roast beef with mustard or salsa
- Half an avocado with raw vegetables
- One or two soft or hard boiled eggs
- Tomato slices with fresh sliced mozzarella cheese drizzled with olive oil and basil
- One piece of fresh fruit (no canned), low on the Glycemic Index such as grapefruit, orange, apple, berries, melon, pear, cherries, grapes, plum, peach, and nectarine
- 2–3 small squares of dark chocolate over 70% cacao, about $^1/_2$ to 1 ounce of chocolate. (Choose this snack once per day.)

TERRY'S PLAN TO STAY FIT

I have personally experienced the benefits of intense, short burst exercise. In my 12–20-minute exercise program, I primarily use a series of kettlebell swings and a stationary recumbent bike.

I use either a 44- or 53-pound kettlebell or do a kettlebell swing 30–35 times, which takes about 60 seconds and is like running 200 meters as fast as you can. I then do a two-minute rest (active) following the intense burst of activity. My two minutes of rest is usually at the lowest level on a recumbent bike.

I call this active rest. This is to provide continued circulation of the blood and to remove lactic acid from the muscles. Depending on your level of fitness, you can start with a 5-pound kettlebell or whatever is most suitable. Women will find the 5- or 10-pound kettlebell more than enough. Men may want to do 20 or 30 pounds for a good exercise regimen.

1. **KETTLEBELL SWINGS:** 60 seconds to full exertion
2. **ACTIVE REST:** Two minutes
3. **REPEAT SEQUENCE** of exertion and active rest for 12–20 minutes

Even if you can only begin exercising and doing kettlebell swings using a 5-pound weight, that would be a good place to start and progressively increase your intensity. You want to continue doing the swing until you run out of breath and then take a two-minute rest. Repeat this sequence five or six times, or as long as it takes to do in a period of 12–20 minutes. Some people do the kettlebell swing for 30–35 swings, and then for their rest period they jump rope for two minutes. I can't for the life of me jump rope so I use the recumbent bike as an active rest period. It is never a good idea to sit down for your rest period. You want to continue moving. You can even just walk around or bounce on your feet.

When the kettlebell swing is done correctly and over a sufficient period of time, every muscle in the body is working. (See the resources listed below for instructions.) The whole idea is to exercise for 20–30 seconds at your highest level of intensity.

A WORKOUT FOR EVERYONE

I think everyone can find 12–20 minutes two or three times a week. In one of Dr. Sears' most severe cases, he worked with a lady who started off walking for 45 seconds and then rested two minutes and walked an additional 45 seconds and continued this process. Altogether, she lost over 60 pounds with nice muscle tone and was in much better health.

Remember, you are only competing against yourself, so work as hard as you can at some form of exercise for 20–30 seconds. For me it's the kettlebells. For others it may be sprinting or swimming 100 yards as fast as you can with a two-minute rest. Repeat until you have your 12–20 minutes in.

I believe everyone can do this. I challenge you to use this menu plan and exercise program for a minimum of six months, and watch the unbelievable results you'll achieve.

Here are a few websites you should explore so you can learn more about high intensity interval training and kettlebell workouts:

Al Sears, M.D.:
alsearsmd.com

Kettlebell Movement:
kettlebellmovement.com

Dragon Door:
dragondoor.com

Search Beginner Kettlebell Routine at
fitnessblender.com

CHAPTER 8
Know How to Find the Right Choice

From Terry Lemerond:
I've spent more than 45 years in the field of natural health. It has changed my life and I know it will change yours.

Let me give you a little bit of background:

> When I was a young man, I loved soda and candy and, like many young people. I had a very unhealthy diet and it showed. In my early 20s, at 5'7" tall, my weight had ballooned to 250 pounds. It took being in the Marine Corps to change my diet and my attitude. With a "strongly encouraged" exercise regimen (a daily obstacle course and a 10-mile run), I became healthier. Healthy eating and regular exercise changed my life profoundly.

I became a lifelong student of natural health and eventually this became not only my passion, but my profession.

I've worked more than 50 years to formulate and introduce hundreds of effective, natural medicines to America. I've been the owner of health food stores and created nutritional manufacturing companies.

During my years in natural medicine, I've traveled the world, spoken with growers, researchers and practitioners, and tried to absorb as much of their knowledge as possible. Along the way, my own health and the health of others with whom I've shared this information has improved. It has been a wonderful experience.

The lifestyle I adopted all of those decades ago in the Marine Corps brought me to where I am today— healthy, at an appropriate weight and with a deeper understanding of health and nutrition. In this book and others, I am sharing my knowledge and experiences with you. I hope it will help you change your life.

Now back to Hintonia, my latest passion, offers what I believe is a cure for the disease that has wracked the Western world.

As I've noted before, *Hintonia latiflora* has been well studied and found to support healthy blood sugar validated by over 60 years of German research.

This research confirms that Hintonia:

- Maintains blood glucose balance throughout the day
- Supports healthy, natural insulin levels
- Maintains healthy HbA1C levels (long-term blood sugar levels)
- Normalizes carbohydrate metabolism

WHAT TO LOOK FOR

A Hintonia product with vitamin and mineral support is best. I like one that includes a variety of B vitamins (thiamin, riboflavin, B6, B12, biotin and folate), vitamins C and E, and the minerals zinc and chromium. Small amounts of other nutrients as a baseline of vitamin and mineral support were used in the clinical studies on this formula. All have been clinically proven to help achieve and maintain healthy blood sugar levels.

Look for a product that has all of the above plus 100 mg of *Hintonia latiflora* standardized for 20 mg polyphenols per dose. If you have mild to moderate diabetes, you'll need to take 2-3 capsules daily to get blood sugars under control. One of the amazing aspects of *Hintonia latiflora* is it will not take your blood sugar too low, so you don't have to worry about becoming hypoglycemic.

I recommend starting with two capsules per day for lowering elevated blood sugars. Some patients have noted dramatic declines in HbA1c levels—as much as an impressive dramatic drop from 14.1 to 6.0 in a month!

Even a small reduction in A1C can have huge benefits for our health and wellness. A one percentage point decrease in A1C can lead to a 25% reduction in microvascular (the smallest blood vessels in our body), 19% reduction in risk of cataracts, 16% reduction in risk of heart failure, and 43% less risk of amputation or death from peripheral vascular disease.

Additionally, *Hintonia latiflora* has side benefits rather than side effects. Research has shown it may help stop gastrointestinal damage and gastric ulcers. Considering the harsh digestive system effects of some drugs used for type 2 diabetes, this is yet another reason to keep Hintonia in your daily diabetes-fighting regimen.

Whether you have elevated blood sugars or full-blown type 2 diabetes, give Hintonia a try. I know you won't regret it.

CHAPTER 9
Doc-to-Doc

Dear Doctor,

Let me introduce myself: I am Jacob Teitelbaum, MD, an integrative physician, author, and health consultant based in Hawaii. I have invited your patient to share this information with you because I think it can be very helpful in helping those you treat.

The prevalence of diabetes and its cousin, metabolic syndrome (diabetes/insulin resistance, hypertension and elevated cholesterol), is skyrocketing. It is estimated that as many as 50% of Americans will develop diabetes or prediabetes during their lifetime.

It is sobering to realize that adult-onset diabetes was once extremely rare until just a couple of decades ago. This suggests that it relates to multiple factors of modern life. It also suggests that it is preventable and treatable.

Although insulin is lifesaving for Type 1 diabetes, using it in Type 2 diabetes often results in severe weight gain with secondary worsening of insulin resistance. So although this therapeutic "loan shark" may be necessary for acutely elevated blood sugars, it is very problematic in the long term for Type 2 diabetes with insulin resistance.

In addition, except for metformin, most diabetes medications have been shown to be more toxic than beneficial. Sadly, in my 40 years as a physician, this research routinely seems to not be given much attention until each medication's patent runs out.

Because of this, it is helpful to have other alternatives that augment our therapeutic arsenal. There are a number of these, but I would like to invite you to consider a very safe, low cost and effective herbal treatment called *Hintonia latiflora.*

WHAT IS HINTONIA LATIFLORA?

Hintonia is an extract of the bark of a shrubby tree that grows in the Sonoran desert. It has been used in folk medicine in Mexico and Central America to treat and even reverse high blood sugar, insulin resistance, type 2 diabetes, and metabolic syndrome for over a century.

It's been studied in detail for its ability to reverse high blood sugars for the past 60 years.

After a number of case reports showing efficacy, 10 more studies have been published looking at this herb's effectiveness in treating diabetes.[1–10] Research has shown that it was so effective that many patients with Type 2 diabetes could reduce or eliminate their need for insulin, especially those needing 25 units a day or less.[1] They were also routinely able to lower the dose or eliminate their oral hypoglycemic agents.[2-10]

Both animal and in vitro studies also confirm this effect while demonstrating multiple underlying mechanisms of action.[11-13]

To give an idea of its effectiveness, one *Hintonia latiflora* study[2] followed 177 patients with prediabetes or mild Type 2 diabetes for eight months. Patients consumed capsules that included Hintonia as the primary ingredient. During the study, patients were evaluated every two months on various parameters of diabetes, including HbA1C, fasting glucose and postprandial blood sugar, as well as common symptoms associated with diabetes, such as neuropathy. At the end of eight months, researchers noted the following significant improvements:

- HbA1C improved by a significant average of 10.4 percent (a ~ 1% drop in HbA1C)
- Fasting glucose improved an average of 23.3 percent
- Postprandial glucose decreased by an average of 24.9 percent

Improvements were also found in diabetic symptoms, as well as blood pressure, cholesterol and liver enzyme values.

Hintonia latiflora is an incredibly safe herbal medicine. Researchers followed up with study participants for almost three years, and there were no side effects or any problems taking it in combination with blood-sugar-control medications.

MECHANISMS OF ACTION

1. Hintonia inhibits glucosidases,[12] slowing the breakdown and absorption of sugar in the gut. This delays the release of sugar into the bloodstream and keeps glucose levels low instead of allowing them to spike, a main cause of excessive insulin release.
2. Coutareagenin, a polyphenol nutrient found in the bark extract unique to Hintonia, appears to be responsible for other blood-sugar-controlling benefits of Hintonia. This unique flavonoid has been shown to reduce insulin resistance and inflammation.[13-14]

One of Hintonia's greatest benefits is that it maintains steady blood glucose throughout the day and night, contributing to long-term improvements in glucose control.

The president of the International Diabetes Foundation was the lead author on another study that strongly recommended the use of Hintonia in treating and preventing Type 2 diabetes, largely because of improved blood glucose control, but also because of its effectiveness in lowering cholesterol and triglycerides. It also helps increase vasodilation.[11]

HOW TO USE HINTONIA

The best Hintonia supplement should be standardized to contain at least 20 mg two to three times a day of polyphenols associated with coutareagenin.

Hintonia has only recently become available to the North American public. No side effects or contraindications have been discovered in more than 60 years of research.

Thanks for taking the time to read this chapter. It is my hope that you will find this information helpful in treating those with insulin resistance, including diabetes, prediabetes and metabolic syndrome.

Best wishes,

Jacob Teitelbaum, M.D.

Doc-to-Doc References

1. Kuhr R. Orale diabetestherapie mit einem Eupharbiazeenextrakt. *Der Landarzt.* 1953;29(23):542–49.

2. Schmidt M, Hladikova M. Hintonia concentrate – for the dietary treatment of increased blood sugar values: Results of a multicentric, prospective, non-interventional study with a defined dry concentrate of Hintonia latiflora. *Naturheilpraxis mit Naturmedizin.* February 2014.

3. Korecova M, Hladikova M. Treatment of mild and moderate Type-2 diabetes: open prospective trial with Hintonia latiflora extract. *European Journal of Medical Research.* 2014;19(1):16.

4. Korecova M, Hladicova M, Korec R. Hintonia latiflora bei Typ-2-Diabetes. *Zeitschrift für Phytotherapie.* 2006;27:272–78.

5. 5. Machens R. Therapieversuch mit Copalchi-Rinde bei pathologischer

Glucosetoleranz. *Erfahrungsheilkunde.* 1996;45(9):605–08.

6. Pellegrini A. Klinisches Gutachten über das Hintonia latiflora Produkt. Sonderdruck Fa. Sippel, Konstanz. 1951:1–7.

7. Schmid P. Bericht über die Behandlung mit dem peroralen Antidiabetikum Hintonia latiflora. Sonderdruck Fa. Sippel, Konstanz. 1951: 1–4.

8. Vida F. Erfahrungsbericht mit dem peroralen Antidiabetikum Hintonia latiflora. Med Welt. 1951;20:1623–24.

9. Ritzmann H. Beitrag zur DiabetesBehandlung. Hippokrates. 1950;21(6): 161–68.

10. Cristians S, Guerro-Analco JA et al. Hypoglycemic activity of extracts and compounds from the leaves of Hintonia standleyana and H. Latiflora: potential alternatives to the use of stem bark of these species. *Journal of Natural Products,* 2009 Mr 27:72(3);4-08-13.

11. Vierling, C, Baumgartner CM et al. The vasodilating effect of a Hintonia latiflora extract with anti-diabetic action. *Phytomedicine* 2014 Oct 12:21(12):1582–86.

12. Mata R, Cristians S et al. Mexican antidiabetic herbs: valuable sources of inhibitors of a-glucosidases.

13. Korec R, Heniz Sensch K et al. Effects of the neoflavonoid coutareagenin, one of the antidiabetic active substances of Hintonia latiflora, on streptozotocin-indicted diabetes mellitus in rats. *Arzneimittelforschung.* 2000 Feb;50(2):122–28.

14. Chen J, Mangelinckx S, Adams A, Wang ZT, Li WL, De Kimpe N. Natural flavonoids as potential herbal medication for the treatment of diabetes mellitus and its complications. *Nat Prod Commun.* 2015 Jan;10(1): 187–200.

Research On Hintonia

Chen J, Mangelinckx S, Adams A, Wang ZT, Li WL, De Kimpe N. Natural flavonoids as potential herbal medication for the treatment of diabetes mellitus and its complications. *Natural Product Communications* 2015 Jan;10(1):187–200.

Cristians S, Guerrero-Analco JA et al. Hypoglycemic activity of extracts and compounds from the leaves of Hintonia standleyana and H. latiflora: potential alternatives to the use of the stem bark of these species. *Journal of Natural Products* 2009 Mar 27;72(3):408–13.

Guerrero-Analco J, Medina-Campos O et al. Antidiabetic properties of selected Mexican copalchis of the Rubiaceae family. *Phytochemistry* 2007 Aug;68(15):2087–95.

Korec R, Heinz Sensch K et al. Effects of the neoflavonoid coutareagenin, one of the antidiabetic active substances of Hintonia latiflora, on streptozotocin-induced diabetes mellitus in rats. *Arzneimittelforschung*. 2000 Feb;50(2):122–28.

Korecova M, Hladicova M, Korec R. Hintonia latiflora bei Type-2 Diabetes. *Zeitschrift für Phytotherapie*. 2006;27:272–78.

Korecova M, Hladikova M. Treatment of mild and moderate Type-2 diabetes: open prospective trial with Hintonia latiflora extract. *European Journal of Medical Research* 2014 Mar 28;19:16.

Kuhr R. Orale diabetestherapie mit einem Eupharbiazeenextrakt. *Landarzt*. 1953;29(23):542–49.

Leyte-Lugo M, Figueroa M, González Mdel C Metabolites from the endophytic [corrected] fungus Sporormiella minimoides isolated from Hintonia latiflora. *Phytochemistry* 2013 Dec;96:273-78.

Machens R. Therapieversuch mit Copalchi-Rinde bei pathologischer Glucosetoleranz. *Erfahrungsheilkunde*. 1996;45(9):605–8.
Mata R, Cristians S et al. Mexican antidiabetic herbs: valuable sources of inhibitors of a-glucosidases. *Journal of Natural Products* 2013 Mar 22;76(3):468–83.

Rivera-Chávez J, Figueroa M et al. a-Glucosidase Inhibitors from a Xylaria feejeensis Associated with Hintonia latiflora. *Journal of Natural Products* 2015 Apr 24;78(4):730–35.

Rivera-Chávez J, González-Andrade M et al. Thielavins A, J and K: a-Glucosidase inhibitors from MEXU 27095, an endophytic fungus from Hintonia latiflora. *Phytochemistry* 2013 Oct;94:198–205.

Schmidt M, Hladikova M. Hintonia concentrate—for the dietary treatment of increased blood sugar values: Results of a multicentric, prospective, non-interventional study with a defined dry concentrate of Hintonia latiflora. *Naturheilpraxis mit Naturmedizin*. February 2014.

Vierling C, Baumgartner CM et al. The vasodilating effect of a Hintonia latiflora extract with antidiabetic action. *Phytomedicine* 2014 Oct 15;21(12):1582–86.

About the Authors

Terry Lemerond

Terry Lemerond is a natural health expert with over 50 years of experience helping people live healthier, vibrant lives. A much sought-after speaker and accomplished author, Terry shares his wealth of experience and knowledge in health and nutrition through his educational programs. They include the *Terry Talks Nutrition* website—TerryTalksNutrition.com— newsletters, podcasts, webinars, personal speaking engagements, and his popular, weekly radio show. His books include *Seven Keys to Vibrant Health, Seven Keys to Unlimited Personal Achievement,* and 50+ Natural Health Secrets Proven to Change Your Life. Terry continues to author and co-author books with dedication, energy, and zeal around his ongoing mission — to help everyone improve their health.

Dr. Jacob Teitelbaum

Jacob Teitelbaum, M.D., is one of the most frequently quoted integrative medical authorities in the world. He is the author of the best-selling books *From Fatigued to Fantastic!, Pain Free, 1,2,3!, The Complete Guide to Beating Sugar Addiction, Real Cause Real Cure, The Fatigue and Fibromyalgia Solution* and the popular, free smart phone app *Cures A–Z.*

He is the lead author of numerous research studies and appears often as a guest on news and talk shows nationwide, including *Good Morning America, The Dr. Oz Show, Oprah & Friends, CNN* and *Fox News Health.* Learn more at Vitality101.com.

More about TTN Publishing, LLC

Everyone has the same desire:
a vibrant, healthy life!

TTN Publishing exists to provide educational information anyone can use to understand how herbs and botanical medicines play a vital role in optimal health. From a stomach ache to a life-threatening disease, even cancer, the plant kingdom has safe, effective phytonutrients and answers for healthy living.

Author and health pioneerTerry Lemerond brings his vast knowledge of plant medicines combined with cutting edge research from today's top scientists and doctors directly to consumers.

Each TTN Publishing, LLC book is crafted to provide the necessary basic information and recommendations for how botanicals can be used in practical ways to fight disease and improve the path to healthy living.

Education, information, scientific validation, and common sense are a part of every TTN Publishing endeavor. There are many books to come, so stay connected! With 80 percent of the world's population depending on plant medicines, you can join in the knowledge and wisdom available to meet your health goals.

WELCOME TO TTN PUBLISHING!

We'd love to hear from you!
info@ttnpublishing.com
TTNPublishing.com
Would you like to be one of the first to know the latest updates on Terry's books?

- Learn more about his background and new books
- See photos, videos, and the latest news
- Listen to Terry's radio show, including archived programs on a multitude of subjects
- Sign up for a free weekly email newsletter and educational webinar notices

It's all available at TerryTalksNutrition.com

Don't forget to connect at:
facebook.com/TerryTalksNutrition

- Visit and follow Terry's author page on Amazon -amazon.com/author/terrylemerond

Share your good thoughts with other health seekers and leave a book review!

Share this exciting news!

If you appreciated this book, please let others know.

- Pick up another copy and share with a friend
- Talk about it on social media
- Write a review on your blog or website
- Recommend this book to friends and family

Thank you for being a true health seeker!
TTN Publishing, LLC

Made in the USA
Monee, IL
11 October 2026

65443003R00059